Caring For An Elderly Person At Home

A Friendly Guide

Pearl Whitehead

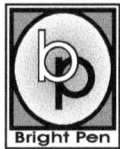

A Bright Pen Book

Text Copyright © Pearl Whitehead 2014

Cover design by © Authors OnLine

All rights reserved. No part of this publication may be reproduced, stored in a retrieval system, or transmitted in any form or by any means, electronic, mechanical, photocopy, recording or otherwise, without prior written permission of the copyright owner. Nor can it be circulated in any form of binding or cover other than that in which it is published and without similar condition including this condition being imposed on a subsequent purchaser.

British Library Cataloguing Publication Data.
A catalogue record for this book is available from the British Library

ISBN 978-0-7552-1648-2

Authors OnLine Ltd
19 The Cinques
Gamlingay, Sandy
Bedfordshire SG19 3NU
England

This book is also available in e-book format, details of which are available at www.authorsonline.co.uk

Do you look after a sometimes awkward, cantankerous and stubborn old person?

I do too, he is my father.

And straight away I find myself slightly upset at having confessed to such thoughts, for I like to think of myself as a good and dutiful daughter. When I am less emotionally affected, I can recognize that there are logical reasons why he sometimes behaves in such a way and for most of the time he is a reasonable, sociable and fun-loving man. And I do love him dearly.

Perhaps you have experienced similar feelings yourself, whether you are caring for a husband, wife, other relation or a friend. If so, this friendly guide to caring for an elderly person at home will help you to cope with the practical, financial and emotional difficulties of caring.

WHY I WROTE THIS BOOK

This book is not a textbook or instruction manual but a friendly guide based on my personal experience of caring for elderly people. Having already produced three books on the training of people who work in homes for elderly people, I feel that much of the information in the books is relevant to people who care for an elderly friend or relative in a voluntary capacity.

It has been my intention to cover some aspects of care, favouring a common-sense approach rather than inflexible correctness. I have tried to moderate the didactic tone associated with training manuals and to adopt a less officious style, inserting some anecdotes drawn from my own experiences. Even so, imparting such a lot of information does require structure, so I have divided the book into broad subject areas and within them written short, detailed paragraphs covering various aspects of caring.

I have used the term 'carer' to mean a friend or relative who is giving the care to an elderly person, without payment. The designation 'care worker' is applied to a paid worker who is required to undertake formal training. The book is not aimed at care workers, childcare workers or carers for people with specific mental or physical disabilities, although some of the contents of the book might be relevant to their area of work. If you are a carer and wish to achieve a formal qualification in care you may wish to investigate the possibility of gaining a BTEC Diploma in Health and Social Care.

For the sake of brevity I have used 'friend' to include any elderly relation or person for whom you are caring.

It has been my intention to write about the common issues of caring for the older person. There are specific aspects of care, such as caring for a person with Alzheimer's disease or looking after a person who has had a stroke, where more detailed information can be obtained from other sources. A friend of mine recently told me that it was the practical details of caring for his wife that caused him most stress, by which I think he meant, feeding and dressing and personal care. I have tried to give thought to such particulars.

And what does old or elderly mean? In my reading for this book I came across a study that defined 'elderly' as somewhere between 60 and 75 years of age and 'old' as beyond those years. After my father's first visit to the local day centre when he was 90, he decided it wasn't for him as all the people there were old. We probably all know of acquaintances who are old at 60 or still young at 90. Much seems to depend on good physical and mental health.

One man of my acquaintance told me that he could pinpoint the exact moment when he became 'old'. It was autumn and after washing his car he set about vacuuming up the leaves on his front lawn. Having picked up the last leaf and looking forward to his coffee break he turned round to admire his work only to find that his still damp car was completely covered by the leaves he had so carefully cleared from the garden. He had forgotten to put the collection bag on the garden vac. He sat down in disbelief and despair. I related this story to my 40-year-old son whose response was that it was the just sort of thing he too, was capable of doing.

Unless we succumb to a stroke or some debilitating disease becoming 'elderly' is a gentle process. We all get forgetful but it will serve us well to remember that the majority of older people need no care at all, while many get by with only a little help from their friends. My 99-year-old father and my **elderly aunt** both live an independent life in their own homes with just a little support from family and friends.

My own children think that my ulterior motive for writing this book is to ensure that they know how I expect to be cared for when I become an elderly person!

NB At this point I am required to state that while a great deal of effort has been made to ensure the information in this book accurate and up to date, the information must not be used as any sort of authority for the way you care for an elderly person.

Since I started writing this book I have had to correct several useful

website addresses and telephone numbers which were correct at the time of writing but have since changed. I cannot guarantee that they will not change again.
PW

A WORD OF THANKS

To my elderly relatives who were included in the narrative and were very amused by their inclusion. To Gwyn Williams who encouraged me to use my experience with elderly people to write this book and who patiently transferred my endless chattering and memories on to paper.

To my husband who was supportive throughout, providing essential supplies of coffee and less essential advice.

To the websites of Age UK, Patient.co.uk, Gov.uk and NHS Choices who provided support when I needed a nudge in the right direction.

CONTENTS

LOOKING GOOD, FEELING GOOD 1

Why is personal care an important issue for your elderly friend?...How you can detect when your elderly friend is neglecting their personal care...You can make personal care easier...Poor hygiene can cause problems...Professional staff can help you provide good care.

WHERE'S THE NEAREST LOO? 6

Urinary incontinence is often a problem for elderly people...There are things that can be done to minimize the embarrassment of being incontinent...Professional help is available.

WHAT'S FOR LUNCH? 9

Why should your elderly friend have a healthy diet?...What is a healthy diet for most people?...What is an unhealthy diet?...Reasons why elderly people may not eat well...Shopping for food...Why do some elderly people find eating difficult?...Suggestions for making eating less difficult...How to encourage your elderly friend to eat...Your choice or theirs?...Food hygiene...Poor food hygiene...Kitchens are hazardous places, especially for elderly people...Adverse reactions to food...Professional help.

GETTING AROUND 17

Why is it beneficial for your elderly friend to stay active?...There are aids available to help people with restricted mobility...Safe mobility around the home...Safe mobility outside the home...How to help your elderly friend stay mobile...Sources of professional help.

TALKING AND LISTENING 23
Verbal communication is about using words….. What is non-verbal communication?..... The main barriers to communication….. Simple ways to help with communication

MONEY, MONEY, MONEY 28
Help available for elderly people….. State Pension….. Pension Credit….. Attendance Allowance….. Personal Independence Payment….. Carer's Allowance….. Winter Fuel Payment….. Help to collect benefits….. Housing Benefits and Council Tax Benefits….. Travel….. Help with gardening….. Power of Attorney

OUT AND ABOUT 34
New technology….. Shopping….. Library….. Interest groups….. Day centres….. Recreational classes….. Pets….. In conclusion

KEEPING SAFE 38
What is meant by abuse?..... Physical abuse….. Sexual abuse….. Financial abuse….. Emotional and psychological abuse….. Neglect….. Discrimination….. How can you tell if your friend is being abused?..... What can you do if you suspect your friend is being abused?

BE A GOOD FRIEND 44
Speak as you would wish to be spoken to….. Treat with dignity….. Respect privacy….. Confidentiality….. Encourage individuality….. Maintaining independence….. Different cultures and values

CARING FOR THE CARER 48
Who is a carer?..... For those of us who are not angels….. People who can help

WHAT HAPPENS NEXT? 51

ABOUT THE AUTHOR 52

LOOKING GOOD, FEELING GOOD

Why is personal care an important issue for your elderly friend?

I take personal care to mean washing and grooming. I suppose we can all tell tales of elderly friends who lived in houses without hot running water and who did not feel the need for frequent changes of underwear. Now, with the advent of washing machines, maintaining personal hygiene has become easier and our standards are by and large higher than generations ago.

Standards of personal care have always varied from one person to another. Some elderly people are quite fastidious, like my aunt and others less so, like my father who thinks cleanliness is a bit overrated! For an elderly person, a bath or shower may take a great deal of effort and they may become reluctant to bother. They may have poor eyesight and/or restricted movement of their limbs, so do not have the confidence to have a bath or shower alone. It may also be that, even if they have sufficient money, they perceive that the cost of heating water, washing and drying clothes puts a strain on their finances.

The consequences of poor personal hygiene and an unkempt appearance are that your elderly friend becomes socially isolated. And here comes a moral predicament, should you try to impose your standards of cleanliness on your elderly friend who may feel that you are being too controlling and particular?

How you can detect when your elderly friend is neglecting their personal care

The signs of losing interest in personal care are many, varied and eventually obvious. The first indication might be the outward appearance of your elderly friend. Facial stubble might be fashionable for young men but elderly men who regularly appear unshaven are inclined to look unkempt. Other signs are unbrushed, uncombed, unwashed or uncut hair, dandruff on the clothes, dirty spectacles, dirty or uncut fingernails and stained clothes. Non-visual indications include unpleasant body odour, bad breath and the smell of stale urine.

You can make personal care easier

If your elderly friend lives alone and lacks confidence in bathing, you may be able to offer help. This could mean just being in the house, or running the bath water or helping them in and out of the bath or shower.

To enable your friend to remain independent, there are all sorts of aids available to make bathing easier. They include grab rails fixed to a wall, a low-entry bath, a swivelling bath seat, a bath lift to lower and raise the bather and a bath stool designed to be placed within the bath. Some people will find it easier to take a shower where they can use grab rails and a perching stool or a chair. Easy to use lever taps can be fitted to wash basins and baths. These adaptations may possibly be supplied through the social service's occupational health department. Other useful aids might be available at a specialist mobility retail outlet. Two elderly acquaintances of mine told me that the most useful item in their bathroom was the bidet!

There are steps you can take to help your elderly friend to maintain good personal hygiene. For instance you may be able to put toothpaste, toothbrushes, combs and hairbrushes within easy reach; introduce the use of a denture pot and denture cleaning tablets; buy lotions, oils, gels, talcum powder and perfumes to make bathing a pleasant experience; buy wet wipes or liquid soaps to make hand washing easier and alcohol wipes to make cleaning spectacles easier. When shaving is becoming difficult suggest a magnifying mirror or even offer to help.

Hair care is important. Scalp skin, just like any other skin on the body, must be kept clean. Shampooing should be done at least weekly as oils build up on the scalp and may cause scalp irritation. Long, untidy hair gives one a dishevelled appearance. For women and men a regular visit to the hair salon can become a highlight of the week or month. Ladies may enjoy the pampering of the beauty therapist for a pedicure, a manicure or a head or foot massage. These treatments are not free but are good for morale.

Make dressing easier for your elderly friend by arranging their clothing in drawers and cupboards where they can be easily reached. Lay out clothes, socks and underwear in the evening ready for dressing in the morning. Encourage them to wear clothes that require washing rather than dry cleaning and to purchase non-iron clothes and permanent crease trousers. Clothes that fasten at the back or which have too many buttons, such as shirts and blouses, can make dressing difficult. Consider using T-shirts, polo necks and clothing with zips or elasticated waistbands, which are easier to use than buttons. Velcro fastening shoes and slippers are easier to manage than lace-ups. Many older men prefer to wear soft-top socks for comfort.

Not all of these aids will be appropriate for helping the person for whom you are caring and a visit to an outlet that sells disability aids may prove worthwhile. Ask to see aids that are appropriate for the specific problems faced by your friend.

Poor hygiene can cause problems

Good hygiene is not just about looking and smelling pleasant. Poor personal hygiene can result in physical problems including poor mobility caused by lack of foot care and eating difficulties due to poor dental care. Social consequences include poor self-esteem and loss of social contacts.

My father initially resisted the idea of me bathing him and washing his hair every week. He obviously felt it to be an invasion of his privacy. The alternative was to leave him to look after his own personal care. As he cannot stand unaided this was a very perfunctory look at a facecloth and a hair wash with a bar of soap which left him with a dandruff problem. He enjoys receiving the visitors who come to see him frequently and I persuaded him that they would not stay long if he neglected his personal hygiene. So I appealed to his vanity and now he looks forward to his weekly bath and reminds me when it is due.

Professional staff can help you provide good care

If you are a carer of an elderly friend you should never feel that it is all too much for you. There are people you can call on for help, such as Age UK and private care agencies. Some local councils have a single assessment process for older people, allowing health and social workers, community nurses and other professional people to share information and act upon it. There will usually be a charge for care services.

Attendance allowance is payable to elderly people to help with paying for these services. (See Money, Money, Money.)

Based on the assessment, social services will provide care workers to help with washing, dressing and making meals. Administering medication, such as eye, ear or nasal drops and collecting prescriptions, is a job for families, but may also be undertaken by carers employed by the social services department. It is possible for a pharmacy, Lloyds is one of them, to provide a weekly monitored dosage system. It is a simple and safe way to take medication and helps those who find it difficult to remember if or when to take their medicines.

Assessments may also be undertaken by an occupational therapist whose job it is to look at an individual's needs and offer appropriate advice. Services they provide include the provision of equipment to help in the home such as mobility aids and tools for preparing meals, washing and dressing and adaptations to the home, e.g. grab rails by the outside door or in the bathroom.

For health care needs the first port of call should be your elderly friend's doctor. He/she can make referrals to the district nurse for wound assessment and care, acute and chronic disease management and palliative and terminal care.

A podiatrist or chiropodist is a professional person who deals with foot care. The care includes treatment of dermatological and other foot related problems such as corns, calluses, verrucas, ingrowing toenails and fungal infections. They also manage foot problems caused by arthritis or diabetes. The service is available both through the National Health Service via a doctor or directly by a private practitioner.

Physiotherapy can help people who have a degree of incontinence, heart problems, breathing difficulties, arthritis or who have had a stroke. This service is available through the NHS or a private practice as is dental care.

Information and contact details about services that can be provided can be found on your local council's website, or through leaflets provided at the council's offices. You can also search for your local council on the Gov.uk website. Libraries often have the same information available. Alternatively, you may find your friend's doctor will be able to help with a referral to the services required. Be aware that if you use a private practice there will be a charge.

WHERE'S THE NEAREST LOO?

Urinary incontinence is often a problem for elderly people

Continence is the ability to control the bladder. Urinary incontinence is the unintentional leakage of urine from the bladder. It affects both men and women. If you suspect that your elderly friend has become incontinent, encourage them to visit their doctor for advice.

Stress incontinence occurs suddenly when there is pressure on the lower stomach muscles, e.g. when coughing, sneezing or laughing. It is aggravated if an individual is overweight as there is then more pressure on those muscles.

Urge incontinence is when you feel an urgent need to pass urine but are not able to reach the toilet in time. An enlarged prostate gland is quite a common condition in older men that creates pressure on the bladder and the urethra. This results in incontinence or the need to pass urine frequently. Again, being overweight puts additional stress on the abdominal muscles and weak abdominal muscles can result in poor bladder control. Poor mobility might exacerbate the difficulties of an individual who has slight continence difficulties. It might be that a person can respond to the need to go to the toilet but cannot get there in time because the toilet is too far away. Mobilizing with sticks or a walking frame may be too slow and restricted arm movements may make the removal of underwear difficult.

Drinking a lot of fluid over a short period of time increases the amount of urine the bladder has to deal with. Not drinking enough fluid causes urine to become concentrated and this will irritate the bladder, making regular visits to the toilet a necessity. Alcohol, teas, coffees and carbonated drinks, even without caffeine, can cause the kidneys to produce more urine. Alcohol also can impair the ability of the individual to recognize the need to urinate.

There are things that can be done to minimize the embarrassment of being incontinent

Some older people become distressed over their inability to maintain their continence. They see the situation as a loss of dignity, privacy and a serious restriction of a social life. They are anxious about their situation because of the fear of wetting themselves, causing an unpleasant odour or becoming a nuisance to other people with whom they live. Ultimately the fear is that they might not be able to continue to live at home.

There are ways of alleviating the distress and embarrassment of incontinence. You will need to offer assistance and advice with great sensitivity. Allow your friend to talk about their feelings if that is what they want to do, although many will prefer not to do so. Assure them that what they have told you will remain confidential. Support them if they are distressed, by being kind and sympathetic and suggesting ways of dealing with the situation.

Help them to come to terms with changes in their lives by presenting the situation to them in a positive manner. If the main problem is not being able to get to the toilet on time, you can offer advice on a range of clothing that will allow them to undress quickly, for example, trousers with an elastic waist, stockings rather than tights. Think about how you can help them to access the toilet quickly. Toilets can be modified with a toilet frame, or a toilet frame with a seat that can be height adjusted or grab rails can be fitted to an adjacent wall. All of which may help with getting on to the toilet on time. Perhaps if the only toilet is upstairs and there is money available, having a downstairs toilet installed might be a feasible solution. Some might say a commode is a solution, but to me it solves one problem by creating three others. Where to put it, where to empty it and by whom?

Advise your friend that the use of incontinence pads will reduce the anxiety and discomfort of wet underclothes. The pads are readily available, disposable or reusable, in a variety of shapes and sizes from the local pharmacy or a disability living outlet. A limited range will be provided free of charge from the district nursing service. There are also many different types of washable fabrics that can be used on duvets, pillows, mattresses and chairs to prevent contamination by urine.

You may need to consult your local authority about the disposal of used inco-pads but generally, incontinence pads do not require a clinical waste collection and can be double bagged and placed in the bin with your household waste, but never down the loo.

Professional help is available

You can find professional help in dealing with incontinence from several sources. A doctor will be able to carry out an assessment and prescribe medication if it is needed, offer advice and refer you to the district nurse, physiotherapist or occupational therapist.

A district nurse will offer help and advice on the range of free incontinence aids available. The physiotherapist can teach individuals to do exercises to strengthen their pelvic floor muscles in order to improve the control of passing urine. The occupational therapist can provide aids and equipment such as raised toilet seats, grab rails and arm rests in toilets to make it easier to go to the toilet.

Further information on continence care can be obtained from organizations such as The Continence Foundation, which produces a range of leaflets and fact sheets, and has a useful website at www.continence-foundation.org.uk

WHAT'S FOR LUNCH?

Why should your elderly friend have a healthy diet?
The answer is because an unhealthy diet is a risk factor of heart disease, cancer and age-related diseases such as osteoporosis. Along with other causes it also may contribute to tiredness, depression, anaemia, infection, muscle weakness, poor mobility and poor skin condition.

What is a healthy diet for most people?
A healthy diet is one that is balanced, which means it contains foods from all the major food groups over a period of one to two days. If your elderly friend has a specific health problem, the doctor or dietician might have prescribed a special diet.

Fruit and vegetables are one of our main sources of vitamins and minerals, which the body needs to perform a variety of functions well. For instance, vitamin A helps to strengthen our immune system, B vitamins help us process energy from food, vitamin D helps us maintain healthy teeth and bones and vitamin C helps to keep cells and tissues healthy. Steamed vegetables will maintain a higher proportion of vitamins than boiled or fried vegetables. Fruit and vegetables also contain high amounts of fibre, which helps to maintain a healthy gut and digestive system.

Starchy foods, also known as carbohydrates, are from where we get most of our energy. Our bodies convert these foods into glucose, which is used as energy either immediately or stored for later use. Starchy foods such as potatoes, bread, cereals, rice and pasta should make up about a third of the food we eat. Where you can, choose wholegrain varieties, or eat potatoes with their skins on for more fibre.

Dairy products are great providers of calcium, these include milk, butter and cheese. The most common mineral in the body, calcium, is needed for helping blood to clot, and to keep bones and teeth healthy. Meat, fish, eggs and pulses also provide us with significant amounts of protein, which is essentially a building block of the body. Everything from our hair, muscles, nerves, skin and nails needs protein to build and repair itself.

Fluids are also vital to help our bodies perform their functions effectively, and the best fluid of all is water. It is necessary to help our blood carry nutrients and waste around the body. About six to eight drinks a day is a good average amount. All drinks count, but water, milk and fresh fruit juices are the healthiest.

What is an unhealthy diet?

For the purpose of this section I think that an unhealthy diet is one that contributes to the ill health of an elderly person. For example, a poor diet for a person who is seriously overweight would be a high calorie intake, while for a person who is underweight a poor diet would be one that is low in calories. For most other elderly people a poor diet would include the consumption of an insufficient amount of food and fluids, an insufficient intake of fruit and vegetables and a low intake of meat and fish and an excess of alcohol.

Reasons why elderly people may not eat well

Some elderly people find it more difficult to adhere to a healthy diet because of failing physical or mental health. They may be too tired or unmotivated to cook and so find it easier to eat snack foods rather than to prepare nutritious meals. Poor dental health may restrict what they can actually eat or medication may diminish their appetite. Restricted mobility may affect their ability to stand in the kitchen to cook or go out and shop for food.

Shopping for food

Your elderly friend may not be short of money but perceives that food prices are too high compared with what they remember from the past. For example my father's reaction when I brought home his shopping was to exclaim, "What, that's ten shillings for an orange!" We should bear in mind that £20 for a small bag of shopping was at one time far more that an average person's wages for a week's work. Twenty pounds per week is approximately one thousand pounds a year. I recall my husband first earning that amount of money in the 1960s and I thought we were rich.

When buying or cooking food for an elderly friend remember that if they are reasonably well for their age, they have reached that position with their established diet and there is no necessity to try to change it. However where an elderly person has been given a prescribed diet for an illness, such as obesity or diabetes, help them to maintain the diet by shopping for food that encourages them to adhere to the diet.

My father was brought up in poverty on an excess of bread and potatoes. Although he now eats what I consider to be a good diet he does add a large amount of salt to his dinner and three heaped teaspoonfuls of sugar to his tea. If I remark on it he says, "I'm ninety-nine, what are you telling me?"

Why do some elderly people find eating difficult?

Eating might be a problem because of the physical difficulty or discomfort of managing the eating process. For example, trying to eat quickly or putting too much food on the fork or spoon may cause a problem with chewing or swallowing. Pain or discomfort on eating might be due to a stomach disorder. An inability to chew may be a dental problem caused by mouth ulcers or ill-fitting or simply worn down dentures. When I was managing a nursing home I remember a new arrival told me that she could only eat food that did not need chewing because her false teeth were loose. This is by no means an unusual cause of difficulty for older people. Medication may alter the taste of food or depress the appetite. Limited hand or arm movements may make eating laborious and necessitate the use of special crockery or cutlery.

Suggestions for making eating less difficult

Older people, who have difficulty manipulating standard crockery and cutlery, may benefit from a wide range of alternatives that may be available to borrow from the social services occupational therapy department or to buy from retailers. Crockery available includes two-handled cups for individuals who are unable to control a cup with one hand and beakers with spouts for individuals who cannot properly control the flow of fluid from a cup. Partitioned bowls and plate guards are useful for people who have difficulty putting food on to a fork or spoon.

Further help can be obtained by the use of specially adapted cutlery such as broad-handled knives, forks and spoons and contoured plastic sleeves in different shapes that can be slipped on to cutlery handles to make them easier to grip. If the problem is with restricted hand or arm movements, angled knives, forks and spoons or combination cutlery may be a solution.

Other useful products include protective clothing and non-slip trays. Non-slip plate mats might be appropriate for the use of anyone who needs to push hard to put food on to a fork or a spoon. The amount of assistance and encouragement your friend may require can vary throughout the day according to how well or how tired they are feeling.

How to encourage your elderly friend to eat

You or I may have a good idea of what constitutes a healthy diet but it may not coincide with the wishes and preferences of your elderly friend. You can advise or persuade but you cannot impose your wishes without compromising the right of the elderly person to make their own choices about what and how they eat and where and when they take their meals.

My father says that he eats porridge and a slice of toast every morning; but I can see by the amount of bread and porridge oats left in the cupboard and the absence of crumbs around the toaster that this is not always so. Later he told me he lied to stop me worrying about him. Now I try to make mealtimes a social occasion by staying with him if possible, while he eats his meal, eating with him or inviting him to my house for dinner.

It is important that food is presented in an attractive manner in order to encourage your friend to eat. Make mealtimes an enjoyable experience. Ensure that cutlery is clean with no traces of old food particles between the prongs of forks or stains on the blades of knives and in spoons. Do not use chipped or cracked crockery and glassware. Condiments, sauce containers and sugar bowls look more attractive if they are clean and free of congealed food.

When serving the food ensure that it is attractive to look at. A large plate full of food can be disconcerting whereas smaller portions, well presented, may well be more appealing. Place the portions of food separately on the plate, not in an unappetizing heap; ensure that food is served at the right temperature and that portions are sufficient for the preferences of your friend. If they are reluctant to make or eat a cooked meal, several small snack meals throughout the day might be more acceptable. Such meals can be nutritious and could include soup, poached egg, beans or sardines on toast, ham or chicken sandwich, cheese and biscuits and fresh fruit that is easy to peel and eat, such as apples, pears, grapes, bananas and other fruit in season.

Your choice or theirs?

Allow your elderly friend to make their own decisions about what and how much they eat and drink. As far as is possible allow them to choose their own meal times and the place to eat. Ideally meals should be taken while sitting upright at a table in order to aid digestion. They should be able to spend as long as they wish to eat their meals. If they have a medical condition that requires a special diet, they may need help and encouragement to adhere to it.

Food hygiene

When preparing food for your elderly friend, you might encounter situations where their values in relation to hygiene differ significantly from your own. Unless you think that standards of hygiene threaten the health of the elderly person I feel that you should not interfere.

On the other hand if you feel that the conditions are a risk to their health, you can inform them of the hazards that exist through poor hygiene in the kitchen and advise them of the consequences. Encourage hand washing after using the toilet and if this is becoming difficult for them to do, consider introducing antibacterial hand wipes as an alternative.

Without being heavily prescriptive I suggest that there are some basic guidelines that you might encourage them to follow. Keep food preparation surfaces clean and free from debris that might attract flies, cockroaches, mice and other vermin and discourage pets from being allowed on tables or work surfaces. Persuade them to use hot water for washing crockery and utensils and to keep fresh food covered or refrigerated.

Poor food hygiene

The body's reaction to ingesting contaminated food is commonly known as food poisoning and elderly people are particularly susceptible to it. Symptoms include vomiting, nausea, diarrhoea and stomach pains. All people will not have the same reaction after eating the same infected food and the effects might not be felt until several hours after eating the food.

Kitchens are hazardous places, especially for elderly people

Accidents to people in their own homes are quite common and the most vulnerable groups are older people and young children. One of the accident black spots is the kitchen. Probably the accidents happen to the elderly partly because of their deteriorating eyesight, weak manual dexterity, poor mobility or failing memory. You might be able to identify obvious hazards, which you can either reduce or remove for your friend.

Ideally kitchen floor surfaces should be non-slip with no loose mats that might cause them to trip and you could perhaps check that your friend's shoes or slippers fit properly. Consider replacing a difficult to use tin opener with a new, easy to use and safer model. To help avoid burns and scalds, an oven hob can be made safer by the fitting of a guard rail to prevent a saucepan or frying pan slipping off the top or an elderly person touching a hotplate.

In order to reduce the risk of fire and gas inhalation in his kitchen I persuaded my father to buy a cooker with a hinged lid that turned off the gas supply to all the rings when it was lowered to the hob.

Adverse reactions to food

It might be useful to have some understanding of why some foods cause reactions in certain individuals.

The most common adverse reaction to the intake of food is indigestion. Acid from the stomach irritates the lining of the throat, the stomach or the small intestine. It is the term used to describe a pain or a feeling of discomfort in the upper part of the abdomen beneath the rib cage or a burning sensation in the throat. There are propriety medicines to relieve the symptoms but people suffering from persistent attacks of indigestion should be seen by a doctor.

Food intolerance such as lactose intolerance may be caused by the lack of a specific digestive enzyme or by food additives or preservatives. People will have their own intolerance to particular foods. The caffeine in tea, coffee or chocolate can cause tremor, migraine or palpitations. Red wine and yeast extract can also cause adverse reactions. Symptoms usually occur several hours after eating the food and include headache, abdominal pain, nausea or vomiting, diarrhoea, rashes and palpitations. Generally people will know which foods to avoid and will replace them with suitable alternatives.

Food allergy is a serious condition. The symptoms are related to the individual's immune system. The most common food allergies in adults are to fruit such as strawberries and citrus fruits, vegetables such as celery, onion and to tomatoes, nuts and seafood. Common bodily reactions indicating that a person is allergic to food he/she has eaten include tingling of the tongue or mouth, swelling of the lips, mouth, face, tongue; wheezing, nasal congestion or trouble breathing; abdominal pain, nausea, vomiting or diarrhoea and red blotches on the skin (hives) or itching. If your friend experiences any of these symptoms shortly after eating, seek medical assistance straight away.

Professional help

There are many health professionals whose services you can call upon for help with any eating problems. The first person to call is the doctor who can direct you to the services provided by the National Health Service and the social services of your local authority. They include a dietician who can discuss or adjust a diet, a physiotherapist who may be able to help in cases of muscular weakness or an occupational therapist who may be able to provide eating aids.

Other professionals that you can call upon include a dentist to rectify problems with gums, teeth or dentures and an optician for a client having trouble identifying food on the plate. Emotional problems surrounding eating might benefit from the help of a psychiatrist or counsellor.

GETTING AROUND

This section deals with the importance of older people being mobile, the consequences of becoming immobile and the aids and support available for maintaining mobility. It does not include the care of elderly people who are confined to bed nor does it include the moving and handling of people and heavy objects.

Why is it beneficial for your elderly friend to stay active?

A person who stays physically active is more likely to stay independent for longer than someone who is not physically active. Exercise can make a person feel stronger and more confident with a greater sense of well-being. It might also improve the likelihood of maintaining or reaching a healthy weight, improving sleep and increasing vitality.

Among older adults, falls are a common cause of injury and disability. Physical activity makes bones and muscles stronger. When their muscles are strong, older people are less likely to fall and if they do, they are less likely to break a bone. Age UK says evidence has shown that if elderly people take part in exercise programmes specifically designed to improve strength and balance, the risk of them falling is reduced by half.

Regular physical activity is also good for the brain. Studies have shown that people who do simple exercises, for example, walking briskly, on a regular basis are better able to make decisions than people who aren't physically active. Most older people maintain their mobility through the normal activities of daily living such as shopping, cleaning, gardening or taking the dog for a walk.

Keeping active reduces the risk of developing heart disease, type 2 diabetes, osteoarthritis and osteoporosis. Inactivity plus poor diet can put older people at greater risk of these diseases.

Heart disease occurs when there is a build up of fatty substances in the coronary arteries. It affects more men than women and the chances of getting it increases with age. It is associated with inactivity, high cholesterol and obesity.

Type 2 diabetes occurs either when the body doesn't produce enough insulin to function properly, or when the body's cells don't react to insulin. The risk of developing it increases as you get older. This may be due partly to reduced physical activity on retirement from regular work and the tendency to put on weight at this period.

Osteoarthritis can be found in more than half the people over 65. Bones are thickest and strongest in early adulthood. As you get older your bone density decreases so that bones may become weaker and fragile. It is more common in women than men and mainly affects joints such as knees, hips and fingers.

There are aids available to help people with restricted mobility

If your friend has difficulties with mobility their doctor can refer them for an assessment by an occupational therapist who will have access to a variety of aids and adaptations.

The occupational therapist will initially assess the home environment, and look at any problems your friend may have, including accessing and using the bath or shower, reaching and manipulating kitchen utensils and equipment and washing and dressing.

Many older people negotiate themselves around the house by holding on to the furniture, but there are aids available to help them. The occupational therapist will be able to offer advice and possibly supply some of the aids. There are many variations of the walking stick including the traditional wooden, the lightweight metal, the telescopic and the folding. All of them, except the wooden one, can be adjusted to take account of the height of the user. To provide a greater sense of security a person may prefer a tri or quad stick. A walking frame that is height adjustable, has four legs and is available with or without wheels, is a useful aid. They can all be used indoors and outdoors and often have baskets, bags or trays attached to them.

For people who cannot walk a self-propelling wheelchair will give them mobility. Using a wheelchair indoors might require making adaptations to the home, such as replacing steps with ramps, and removing obstructions, such as rugs and possibly some furniture.

Grab rails by the outside door, half steps and ramps will aid access to or egress from the house. Many people now use electric scooters to give them greater freedom and independence outside the home. Swivel seats are available from mobility shops and are a great help for getting in and out of a car.

Not all of these aids will be appropriate for helping your friend and a visit to a shop that sells disability aids might prove worthwhile.

Getting up and downstairs for some people is a problem. Before getting a stairlift fitted my father used to get up the stairs on his hands and knees and come down on his bottom, one step at a time. Without any aids he found this to be the safest way of negotiating the stairs. Most people of course, now know about stairlifts, whereby you can sit on a seat and press a button to go up and down the stairs. It operates at a safe but slow rate.

There are a variety of different types of chair available to assist a person who has difficulty sitting in or getting out of a conventional chair. A high-backed wing chair can help to maintain a person in an upright position and also to support the head and neck. A chair with a high seat allows a person to rise more easily from the sitting position. A rise and recline chair allows a person a safe way of getting in and out of the chair from and back to a standing position.

Safe mobility around the home

Elderly people are more susceptible to falls than any other group of adults and they tend to be more seriously physically and emotionally affected by them. They are also more likely to break a bone as a consequence of a fall. Accidents can often reduce their confidence, leading to decreased social interaction and increased dependence on other people.

As a carer you can help to reduce the risk of your friend falling by drawing attention to hazards within the home and possible unsafe practices. There may be trailing electrical wires from the television or electric blanket or from a table lamp. Rugs and doormats might be a potential hazard, or walkways obstructed by furniture such as the corners of tables or occasional chairs. There is a risk that elderly people might trip, slip or fall over such obstacles. Poor lighting, particularly in the hall and on the staircase, contributes to accidents. A simple solution is to increase the wattage of the electric light bulbs.

On occasions I have found my father wandering around the house at dusk, in the semi-darkness, without the electric lights on. Putting them all on time switches seemed to solve the problem.

Check the safety of the garden, where hosepipes, garden tools, footpaths and even overhanging trees and bushes all have the potential to be hazardous for a person with poor mobility.

Safe mobility outside the home

The Equality Act 2010 gives disabled people important rights of access to everyday services without discrimination or harassment. Providers of services have an obligation to make reasonable adjustments to their premises or to the way they provide a service. They include libraries, health centres, shops, cafes, banks, cinemas and places of worship. Sometimes it just takes minor changes to make a service accessible to a wheelchair user, such as a ramp or an automatic door.

With the increased availability of mobility scooters, it is possible for your friend to get around the local area independently and enjoy organized activities outside the home. In my experience local tradespeople are very kindly disposed to people with mobility difficulties.

Most supermarkets make extra efforts to try and accommodate people with mobility needs by having wide, unobstructed aisles and in some cases they provide specially adapted trolleys to fit on to wheelchairs and one store that I know of even provides electric powered wheelchairs.

The workers in my father's local store will walk around the shop following him on his mobility scooter, getting for him any items he cannot reach. Of course shopping then becomes a pleasant experience for him because he likes the friendly banter with the staff. In return for their kindness he has offered to take them all on a Caribbean cruise when he wins the lottery!

Try not to allow your elderly friend to be excluded from social and business activities. Think of ways in which their limitations can be accommodated. For example, if possible take them in the car to and from the local social centre.

An acquaintance of mine was having difficulty accessing public transport in her wheelchair. A meeting with the manager of the bus company resulted in a modification of its wheelchair policy, giving wheelchairs priority over pushchairs and wheeled shopping bags. As a result the company displayed appropriate notices at the entrance and exit doors of all of its buses.

Special devices have been designed to make getting into and out of a car easier. Swivel seats are expensive and need adaptations to the car. Much cheaper are swivel cushions that you can place on an existing seat to make that painful twist off the seat much more comfortable. You can buy them from most mobility shops.

How to help your elderly friend stay mobile

You can help your friend to remain active by encouraging them to do their own shopping, cooking and housework as far as they are able to do so.

If they are a car driver or have access to a car and have difficulty walking far, they might be interested in applying to their local authority for a parking concession under the Blue Badge scheme. Applicants will be asked to describe the nature of their disability and give an estimate of the maximum distance they can walk without assistance or severe discomfort. Your local authority may require a mobility assessment with a medical professional, such as a physiotherapist or occupational therapist, in order to determine whether or not they meet the eligibility criteria. For further details of the scheme go to the Internet website http://bluebadge.direct.gov.uk or ask at the local council office.

You can contact the organizers of luncheon clubs or senior citizens' groups and offer to accompany your elderly friend there and pick them up later. Suggest visiting the doctor, chiropodist or optician for appointments, rather than requesting a home visit. By doing so they have a reason for maintaining their mobility and an opportunity for social interaction.

Sources of professional help

If your friend shows signs of difficulty walking due to breathlessness or painful joints encourage them to see their general practitioner who will offer treatment or refer them to one of the health professionals mentioned below.

A physiotherapist may be able to improve co-ordination, muscle strength and posture through movement and exercise or massage to relieve muscle pain and stiffness. Aquatic therapy, which is a form of physiotherapy carried out in water, may be helpful. Other techniques such as heat and acupuncture may be used to ease pain.

An occupational therapist will visit the home and advise on aids and adaptations to assist in daily living activities. They will evaluate the mobility needs of the elderly person, make recommendations and may be able to provide wheelchairs, stairlifts, perching stools, grab rails and other aids to assist in daily activities such as eating, toileting and bathing. The occupational therapist will adjust wheelchairs according to the particular needs of your elderly friend, taking account of the required width of seat, length of footrests, size of wheels (large wheels for hand-propelled chairs) and the possible need for cushioned support.

A chiropodist, sometimes referred to as a podiatrist, will provide care for feet and lower legs. Elderly people sometimes have poor mobility because of foot problems such as corns, calluses, verrucas, infections and ingrowing toenails. Mobility can be significantly improved by treating these conditions.

TALKING AND LISTENING

Effective communication is the cornerstone of good caring. Poor communication can lead to mistakes and misunderstandings. A simple example of this was when my father, after visiting his doctor, told me that he was to take up to eighteen paracetamol tablets a day. In fact the prescription was for no more than eight tablets in a day.

Verbal communication is about using words

It uses speaking, listening, reading and writing skills. The most common ways of communicating are by speaking and listening. Here are some ways in which you can improve your verbal skills.

When speaking, adopt a pleasant, friendly tone of voice. Your tone of voice says as much as the words you use. Speak clearly, loud enough to be heard comfortably and not too quickly. Ask questions to ensure that you have been understood. If your friend has a hearing impairment, stand or sit close to them so they can see your facial expressions and watch your lips. If the conversation is important make sure that there are no distracting noises, e.g. television or radio, and that you can see each other clearly.

In order to communicate well be prepared to listen carefully. You can learn body language techniques that will help you to be a good listener. Face your friend and make eye contact. Adopt an appropriate facial expression and lean slightly forward to show that you are concentrating and wanting to communicate. Say words like, "really", "that's interesting", "of course". Nod the head and show that you have time for listening by sitting in a relaxed manner. Do not keep looking at your watch or fidget. Ask questions to show that you are listening and to give your friend the opportunity to expand on what they want to say.

To encourage conversation ask questions like, "Then what happened?" and "How did you feel?"

To make sure that you and your friend have understood correctly any instructions or arrangements, repeat what you have said and ask questions. For example, when I arranged to take my father to the chiropodist we discussed the time that I should pick him up and before I left his house I asked him to confirm the time he was expecting me.

What is non-verbal communication?

Part of non-verbal communication is popularly known as body language. According to some psychologists, it constitutes over half of the meaning of what we say.

Posture is the way in which we position our body to emphasize what we have to say. It includes how we stand, sit and move around. For example, placing your hands on your hips indicates assertiveness, folding your arms signifies defensiveness and standing up straight shows self-confidence.

Gestures are movements of the body, mainly made with the hands or head, used with or instead of speech to express meaning, intention or feeling. For example, nodding or shaking the head denotes agreement or disagreement, a clenched fist shows aggression and drumming with the fingers indicates impatience.

Making eye contact shows that you are paying attention and facial expressions reinforce the message you are trying to convey, for example, smiling if you wish to reassure someone or serious if passing on important information. If you sit on the edge of your chair and fail to make eye contact with your friend what message are you sending?

Personal space is the space around us that allows us to be comfortable in conversation. It is approximately an arm's length away for all but our close family. We can tell if we are invading our friend's personal space if they lean back or take a step away from us.

How your friend behaves can give you an indication of how they are feeling. Here are some examples. Aggressive behaviour may indicate that they are frustrated or angry. Staying in bed all day or not paying attention to hygiene, dress or appearance might show that they are unhappy or despondent. Becoming unusually quiet and withdrawn and not wanting to participate in their usual social life might indicate that they are distressed or unhappy. Bear in mind that these behaviours might also indicate illness. Sleeping at an inappropriate time or constantly seeking attention may signify boredom. By greeting you in a happy and friendly manner or by participating in the local social life and paying attention to their personal hygiene, dress and appearance, they are indicating a degree of happiness and contentment.

Conversely your friend can make the same interpretation of your behaviour. You will cause confusion if your body language does not match your speech, for example, if you tell a person that something they have done does not matter, while your body is tense and your face expresses anger.

Touching is a form of communication that might be unacceptable to some people while others might accept it as a sign of friendliness and comfort. Some people might consider it unacceptable to be touched on cultural or religious grounds or because touching is not acceptable within the family. To avoid embarrassment and misunderstanding it is advisable to assume that you do not use touch as an aid to communication with your friend until you are sure that it is acceptable. You should be aware that affectionate physical gestures, such as hugging and kissing might be open to misinterpretation. Only through experience will you learn to read your friend's body language and only by knowing them well will you understand if physical contact is acceptable. If in doubt, ask.

The main barriers to communication

Obvious barriers to communication are total or partial loss of hearing, sight or speech. It is also the natural reaction of some people who are emotionally upset, e.g. through the death of a spouse, family disruption, illness or other worries to withdraw from normal social contact.

People with mild confusion may have trouble communicating their needs and they may have difficulty in finding the right word. I consider myself to be a reasonably sensible and sociable person but as I grow older I find that I sometimes have difficulty recalling words, particularly the names of people and places. My friends tell me that they are afflicted in the same way.

As a friend or relative you will probably have sufficient knowledge of the person in your care to understand any cultural, intellectual or social difference that might be the cause of a misunderstanding.

Simple ways to help with communication

There are actions you can take to overcome some of the barriers to effective communication. Partial deafness is quite common among elderly people and can be quite isolating for them. To facilitate conversation with someone who is hard of hearing there should be enough space and light to be seen and quietness to be heard. If they have speech difficulties be patient, sit down and allow them time to speak. If they have a hearing aid, check that it is clean, in good working order, in use and not in their handbag or pocket. If they still have difficulty hearing, you can encourage them to have their hearing aid checked.

To make telephone conversation easier it is possible to buy a specially adapted telephone with a ringer amplifier, flashing light and conversation volume control. You can demonstrate how they can access subtitles on the television. If they have difficulty hearing the doorbell suggest that they could have one installed that has an amplifier and/or flashing light. Some aids can be plugged into sockets, others are battery powered and it may be possible for them to be used anywhere in the house or garden.

If communicating by telephone is a problem, consider exchanging the telephone for one with a large keypad. Perhaps if you can enter the most often used numbers into the quick-dial facility for your friend it will make using the telephone easier.

There are other ways you can help if your friend has failing eyesight. Suggest that they take advantage of audio books and talking newspapers, also possibly books written in Braille. They may be able to access them from their local library service. Most libraries also have a selection of books in large print.

In some areas the fire service provides, free of charge, a fire alarm to put under the pillow in bed. In the event of fire in the night it vibrates to raise the alarm.

If your friend seems to be having trouble with their eyesight and they wear glasses, check that the glasses have been prescribed, do not need to be repaired and are clean. When I visit my father the first thing I do is clean his glasses. I don't understand how he can make them so dirty in a matter of a couple of hours, but he is always pleased when I have done them and he can see clearly again. Ensure that the room is not gloomy and there is plenty of light.

If you are frequently asked to read or write letters for your friend perhaps they might benefit from having an eye test. Most people can have a free NHS eye test every two years if they are 60 years of age or over, and every year if they are 70 years of age or over. (Different rules apply in Scotland.) Elderly people who have difficulty getting to an optician can have an NHS eye test at home; they should not have to pay extra for this service.

MONEY, MONEY, MONEY

Help available for elderly people

Many elderly people are reluctant to ask for financial help and may need persuading to claim for benefits to which they are entitled. If you are caring for an elderly friend and you have reason to believe that they are short of money, they may be eligible for state assistance. However, the benefits, pensions and allowances are many and various and so are the needs and entitlements of individuals. Therefore it is impossible for me to give a definitive assessment of any one person's eligibility for making a claim. It has been estimated by Age UK that every year up to £5.5 billion allocated for Pension Credit, Housing Benefit and Council Tax Benefit, goes unclaimed. You should note that some benefits may affect or be affected by the receiving of other benefits. To add to the confusion the UK government intends to make changes to the benefits system for retired people in the future. Finally you should be aware that the benefits system may be different in Scotland, Northern Ireland and Wales from that which obtains in England.

In a state of bewilderment I set about looking for advice for this section of the book by visiting various government and local government offices in the small town near to where I live. I could not get any leaflets or pamphlets, but it was suggested to me that I could find the information on the Internet. Having trawled through many sites I found that the clearest advice was given by Age UK and I am indebted to that organization for much of the information given below. The Department for Work and Pensions also has a good site and I was also advised that the Citizen's Advice Bureau and charities concerned with the welfare of elderly people could help. What I have attempted to do is give examples in general terms of some of the help that is available. The following paragraphs represent the situation at the time of writing this book.

State Pension

The State Pension age is currently 65 for men and between 60 and 65 for women although the age at which people qualify for a pension will rise in the future. The basic amount payable depends on the National Insurance contributions paid by the individual. A person may qualify for additional payment if he/she has contributed to another state pension scheme.

Pension Credit

Pension Credit is a means-tested benefit for people of pensionable age. It is based on the amount of money that a person has coming in per week and has two parts as follows.

- Guarantee Credit, designed to top-up a pensioner's weekly income to a minimum level of income as set by the government.
- Savings Credit, given if a person has made some savings provision for their retirement.

Pension Credit includes help towards mortgage payments and service charges for homeowners.

Attendance Allowance

If your friend is aged 65 or over and is affected by a physical or mental disability, or perhaps by both, which results in needing assistance with daily living, they might be entitled to Attendance Allowance. To qualify they should be a UK resident and have lived in the UK for at least 26 weeks of the previous year. Assistance with caring means that help is needed with any or all everyday tasks such as, washing, getting into and out of the bath or shower, dressing, eating, getting to the toilet and communicating. The Department for Work and Pensions will decide who qualifies for Attendance Allowance. The money does not have to be used to pay for a carer, but can be spent on whatever the individual decides will help them best. Attendance Allowance is tax-free and is not based on National Insurance contributions, nor is it means-tested (based on income). Attendance Allowance will not adversely affect any other benefits being received, but it may qualify for the receiving of additional benefits. There are two rates of Attendance Allowance to allow for individual circumstances. For further details telephone 0345 6056055.

Personal Independence Payment

PIP is a benefit that replaced the Disability Living Allowance in 2013. A claim for the payment must be made before a person reaches the age of 65. See www.gov.uk/pip

Carer's Allowance

If you are looking after an elderly person, who is living in their own home, you may be able to claim a Carer's Allowance if you spend at least 35 hours a week caring. The allowance is not paid to a person who is under 16 or of pensionable age, in full-time education or earning more than £100 a week. The amount the carer receives depends on the circumstances and the allowance may be affected by any benefits the carer already receives.

See www,gov.uk/carers-allowance/eligibility

Winter Fuel Payment

Most people who are entitled to a Winter Fuel Payment do not need to make a claim. A Winter Fuel Payment should be made automatically to anyone who receives State Pension and/or many other forms of state benefit payment. If this does not happen, you can get a claim form from the Winter Fuel Payment helpline or visit www.gov.uk/winter-fuel-payment

Help to collect benefits

If the person you are caring for is physically incapable of collecting their benefits, you can help to claim or collect them on their behalf if they agree for you to become their appointee. You can only be an appointee if the Department for Work and Pensions has appointed you and you will have to attend an interview.

If your friend receives their payments through a Post Office card account they can apply to the Post Office for one other person to be given permanent access to their account. He or she would be known as a Permanent Agent. In order to use this arrangement the account holder must be capable of managing his or her own affairs.

Housing Benefits and Council Tax Benefits

By applying to the social services of their local authority your friend may be able to get help with Housing Benefit, for example help with paying the rent and Council Tax or, as part of Pension Credit or mortgage interest support. It is a means-tested benefit, so what help they receive depends on their income and savings, with whom they live and how much rent they pay.

Travel

At the time of writing, people over the state retirement age are entitled to free off-peak travel on local buses anywhere in England. Off-peak is generally between 9.30 am and 11.00 pm Monday to Friday and all day at weekends and on public holidays. There may be local conditions such as a charge for the park-and-ride service in York.

If you are of eligible age and you live in Greater London, you can apply for a Freedom Pass. This gives you free travel on the entire London Transport network. On most services, you can use the pass at any time.

Help with gardening

If your friend is finding it difficult to maintain their garden, you might consult your local council for advice or assistance. Some councils offer a garden maintenance service to their council tenants, but to qualify for help an applicant may have to meet certain conditions such as being over 60 years of age, physically unable to do the work and have no other person who is willing and able to help. The council may make a charge for its garden maintenance service.

My father loves gardening and manages to do some whilst leaning over his walking frame with a spade or hoe in his hand. I remember him, when he was in his nineties, digging around the roots of a hedge and blaming the wind when it fell down into his neighbour's garden. He is a son of the soil and seems to believe that everything should be dug over in the winter. However weeding is beyond him apart from the raised flowerbeds and baskets. The rest is my job.

Power of attorney

This section concerns anyone who might wish to act and make decisions on behalf of an elderly person. (I assume that people already holding Power of Attorney will be familiar with their rights and responsibilities.)

Anyone aged 18 or older (to be known as the donor) who has the mental ability to make decisions for themselves can arrange for someone else to make these decisions for them in the future. This can be done at any time. This legal authority is called a Lasting Power of Attorney. The person who is given power of attorney is known as the 'attorney' and must be over 18 years old. The donor can appoint one or more persons as their attorneys and decide how they should act. The granting of a Lasting Power of Attorney is a legal procedure and a person cannot lawfully act as holding a Lasting Power of Attorney unless their application has been registered with the Office of the Public Guardian. To apply you must complete forms that can be obtained from The Office of the Public Guardian, PO Box 16185, Birmingham, B16 6GX, Telephone number: 0300 456 0300.

There are two different types of Lasting Power of Attorney – one covering health and welfare the other covering property and financial affairs. This Lasting Power of Attorney can only be registered and used when the donor is unable to make his or her own decisions.

A health and welfare Lasting Power of Attorney allows the attorney to make decisions for things such as medical treatment. A property and financial affairs Lasting Power of Attorney lets the attorney make property and financial decisions on behalf of the donor. This could include decisions about paying bills or selling a house.

It has been my experience that a person who holds a Power of

Attorney comes under some form of scrutiny, usually informal, from friends or relatives. My advice is to keep clear accounts of transactions that are made by you on behalf of the donor, keeping bills and receipts in a logical filing system. It is good practice to have the transactions vetted by a trusted friend or relative.

The information in this section consists of general advice only and should not be used as an authority for any decision, action or recommendation. The present UK government is undertaking a comprehensive review of state benefits. For up-to-date information contact the Department for Work and Pensions or www.gov.uk/state-pension. I wish to acknowledge my indebtedness to Age UK from which source much of the information in this section is taken.

OUT AND ABOUT

Like most of us, your friend needs a reason for getting up in the morning. Company, entertainment and pastimes may be as important as physical needs. Encourage your friend to keep in touch with their friends and relatives and whenever possible to continue attending any interest groups to which they belong. Some older people, like my father, prefer to socialize outside the home and become low-spirited when on their own for too long. However, my elderly aunt is quite content to pursue her interests in her own home and enjoys the regular visits of the hairdresser, gardener and domestic helper.

Many people retain their independence into advanced old age. Even so, the process of getting old can bring difficulties caused by the deterioration of hearing, eyesight, mobility and memory. Old age might also be a time when someone loses a partner so that they have no one with whom to reminisce or make decisions. Such losses might affect their self-confidence which in turn may lead to isolation and in the worst cases to neglect of their home, garden and themselves.

Here are some suggestions on how to increase the opportunities for your friend to make and keep social contacts and avoid loneliness.

New technology

Think about introducing the idea of staying in touch with friends by using modern technology. A computer, smartphone or tablet, can access social media sites, such as Facebook, Friends Reunited, Skype and Twitter. They can be used to talk to family and friends and to send and receive photographs. Some older people will be resistant to new ideas but my father finds them quite fascinating and is enthusiastic about using them. He has great pleasure in seeing and talking to his great-grandchildren on Skype.

Shopping

Shopping at the local shops is a good way for your friend to meet people and keep in touch with the community. Shop assistants are inclined to be friendly and chat to the customers they see frequently. People who regularly collect their pensions at the post office become well known to the staff. My father is always anxious to collect his money each week when he enjoys a friendly chat with the counter clerk. He is always keen to see the colour of his money, as he is suspicious of banks!

Library

Your local library is often a place where communities meet. It will have large-print books, audio books, DVDs and perhaps a book club. Many libraries are now called resource centres and make provision for free use of computers that allow access to the Internet and online reference facilities. The staff at my local centre are happy to help those who are new to computers and they hold a weekly coffee morning run by volunteers.

Interest groups

If your friend is interested in socializing within a group then it is worth investigating what is available in your area. There may be a senior citizens club that organizes meetings, dances, whist drives, bingo and outings to places of interest. Churches may have activities for the elderly such as coffee mornings, luncheon clubs or fellowship groups. The University of the Third Age (U3A) flourishes in some areas and is specifically for retired people who wish to get together with people who are interested in all sorts of areas. There might be groups for, among other things, gardening, conversational French, painting, reading books and family history. The interested parties choose the activities and most of them take place during the daytime. My sister joined one and started up a group interested in archaeology and my local U3A has a model-making group and a Scottish country dancing group.

Day centres

Day centres for the elderly exist in some areas. The purpose of a day centre is to help prevent social isolation and loneliness among older people. It also provides respite for their relatives and carers. They are run by social services or private companies and may provide various activities including lunch, social events, personal care and advice. There will usually be a charge for attendance.

Recreational classes

Your friend may be interested in learning a new skill or developing one further. My local authority organizes recreational activities such as flower arranging, sugar craft, knitting, costume making, pottery and ceramics, guitar, horticulture, drawing and painting to mention just a few. Your local library, resource centre or U3A may be able to give you information on local groups and activities. Sporting activities are available at local authority or private sports and leisure centres, often with reduced membership fees for senior citizens, and could include suitable activities for older people such as bowls, yoga, aerobics, swimming and aqua fit.

Pets

Small domestic pets can be good company for older people, as caring for them gives purpose to the day and provides companionship and affection. The pets can even provide a reason for turning on the heat to keep the house warm and for preparing a meal. Your friend may find that it is easier to meet and talk to people if they have a dog to take out for a walk. With even the smallest of gardens it is possible to encourage birds on to a bird table or bird feeder, which can provide an interesting diversion.

Outside the patio windows of my aunt's bungalow she has several feeders attracting a wide variety of birds into the garden. She also has a fat ball attached to the end of a long piece of string so that she can pull it into the house if the pigeons start to eat it, as she only likes feeding the little birds!

In conclusion

Try to avoid coercing your friend into activities in order to fulfil your own perceptions of what is right for them. If they do enjoy a good social life you might suggest that they keep track of their appointments and social events by writing notes and using a large calendar or a diary, so that activities do not get forgotten. If, however, your friend is quite shy, it may be that a little help from you is needed in order to encourage interaction with friends and neighbours.

When my aunt moved across the country into her bungalow to be near me, I invited her neighbours in for a drink and mince pies on her first Christmas. She is a very sociable lady within her own home and the neighbours have continued to visit and spend time with her.

Of course not all elderly people need help to socialize. My father seems to be happy working in his garden and driving himself to the Post Office, supermarket or bank on his electric scooter and attending a weekly luncheon club at the local Methodist church. My aunt also seems to be quite content although she rarely leaves her house. She cleans it every day and loves baking cakes, which she gives away to her friends and the birds that congregate at her kitchen door.

KEEPING SAFE

What is meant by abuse?

The whole subject of elder abuse is fraught with misunderstanding and at times presents all sorts of moral dilemmas. Action on Elder Abuse defines abuse as 'a single or repeated act, or lack of appropriate action, occurring within any relationship where there is an expectation of trust, which causes harm or distress to an older person'. The World Health Organization has now adopted this definition. I find it is rather nebulous and so have attempted to give practical examples below under the various types of abuse. Action on Elder Abuse has identified five types of abuse which are physical, psychological, financial, sexual and neglect. However as you will see, it is sometimes difficult to classify a single case of abuse as it may have connections with more than one type of abuse. For example, physical abuse may cause psychological harm. You may have heard of other forms of abuse, such as emotional and discriminatory which could be considered to be part of one of the five types of abuse mentioned above.

An elderly person may be vulnerable to any form of abuse if they become physically frail and/or socially isolated, which make them particularly susceptible to being manipulated or ill treated.

Here are some practical examples of behaviour that might be considered to be abusive.

Physical abuse

Physical abuse is not just hitting, it includes rough, impatient handling such as pulling, pushing and grabbing tightly. This can occur when dressing, undressing or bathing an elderly person or when helping them to move from one position or place to another. Restraining a person is also abusive – it includes removing a walking stick or walking frame to prevent a person from moving around the house. The misuse of medication in order to sedate a person falls into this type of abuse.

Sexual abuse

Sexual abuse of individuals includes the touching of intimate parts of the body without consent and the making of sexual comments, threats or gestures. In order to avoid misunderstanding of your motives it is important to respect and encourage the privacy of an elderly person when they are dressing, undressing, bathing or going to the toilet.

You will probably know your friend well enough to understand if it is appropriate to offer comfort by holding hands or giving them a kiss or a hug, without causing offence.

Financial abuse

After neglect, financial abuse is the most common form of abuse of elderly people. A report by King's College London and the National Centre for Social Research (conducted on behalf of Comic Relief and the Department of Health) concluded that, in one year, at least 57,000 people aged over 66 had experienced financial abuse by a friend, relative or care worker. Financial abuse tends to go hand in hand with increasing age and deteriorating health. According to the King's College study, those living alone or who have care provided for them in their homes are most at risk. They are likely to be the ones who are frail and dependent on others.

Financial abuse of individuals is not just stealing money or possessions. It includes misusing bank books belonging to another person and forging their signature. Influencing a person to part with possessions or money and putting pressure on them concerning the contents of their will is also abuse. If you are involved in spending money on behalf of your friend, it would be wise to keep a record of your transactions to avoid any confusion and to protect you from the accusations from others about how the money has been spent. It would be prudent not to keep a large amount of money that belongs to your friend in your own house. Rather, encourage them to keep their money in the bank.

As so often happens in caring for an elderly person, there is a conflict between your duty to provide protection and the rights of the person to handle their own money. Take for instance my father, who insists on keeping large quantities of money in the house. He has never had a lot of money and he says he likes the feel of it! I have explained why this is not a good idea, but he insists that it is safer than leaving it in the bank! While he is of sound mind and independently spirited I have to accept the situation as it is. He can go to the Post Office and withdraw the money without my knowledge and does not need my permission to keep it where he pleases.

From my experiences of being the manager of a nursing home it was not uncommon for elderly people to mislay their money and declare that it had been stolen. I can assert that I never did find this to be the case and that it was always found amongst the possessions of the elderly person where they had put it for safekeeping. You might like to keep this example in mind should you ever be suspected of theft.

Most people who commit financial abuse are the sons or daughters of the victim. The majority of financial abuse takes place in the elderly person's own home and is likely to occur with the tacit acknowledgement and consent of the elderly person. For example, an elderly person might feel obliged to hand over money to a friend or relation in exchange for their care or friendship.

It is not uncommon for a visitor or distant relative to take an unexpected interest in an elderly person's welfare, wills, inheritance and property. I was surprised recently when I was told by a member of the local police force that abduction of old people from their home by relatives in pursuit of their money, is not an unusual form of domestic incident.

Professional people working in social care are legally bound always to act in the interest of the person receiving care and in accordance with their profession's standards of conduct, performance and ethics. I would expect people who receive no money for their services to behave in a way that protects the financial interest of the person receiving the care. Obviously, all carers remain subject to the laws on theft and fraud.

Financial abuse is often about bringing emotional pressure to bear on an elderly person to part with their money or possessions. It may be a threat (often implied) that they would otherwise lose friendship, care or good will. An elderly acquaintance of mine has a grandson who visits her every week. In spite of having her weekly pension, she has no money for extras for herself and confided to me that she gives all her spare money to her grandson. When I pointed out that perhaps that was not a good idea, as she needed some of that money, she said that the grandson would not visit if she did not give him some money. He was the only member of her family who came to visit her and the only tie with her family, so she chose to be short of money!

Emotional and Psychological abuse

Psychological abuse is the non-physical abuse of a person that causes emotional harm and undermines their self-confidence. It includes threats, humiliation, ridicule, verbal abuse and limiting access to friends and relatives and, in this context, particularly to grandchildren. Here are a few examples of these forms of abuse.

- Telling an elderly person that no one else likes or wants them, that they are fat, ugly and useless, and that they could not manage to look after themselves on their own.

- Forcing them to do things at an exact time or in an exact way.

- Not allowing them to have visitors or controlling who they are allowed to see and who their friends are.

- Not allowing them to be left alone with other people.

- Accompanying them everywhere they go in order to keep control over what they do, who they see and what they say.

Emotional abuse is often difficult to recognize. It can be very subtle, often being overlooked by a person's friends and family. The person affected may not even think or feel that abuse is taking place. It is also closely linked to financial abuse. The abuser makes the older person unnecessarily dependent on them in order to exercise control, but it can damage the self-confidence of the elderly person.

They can be quite vulnerable to this type of abuse as their ability to respond assertively is affected by their need for company and care.

Neglect

Neglect is a form of abuse. It is failure to give appropriate care when it is expected or has been promised and covers a wide range of situations. If neglect occurs as a result of deliberate action then that is abuse. However, if neglect occurs accidentally, say through someone's forgetfulness, that is still abuse according to the definition stated above, as the expected care has not been given. Nearly always such mistakes are not serious and can be rectified.

Discrimination

I am using the word discrimination to mean the unfair treatment of a person because of their race, colour, sex, sexual orientation or religious belief or for any other reason, but particularly in relation to their age.

Elderly people may feel that they are being discriminated against in the provision of medical and social services. For example they may consider that they have been given a low priority on a hospital waiting list, or that other services are not responding to their needs. If you believe that your elderly friend is being discriminated against, you can help to protect them by acting as a go-between, accompanying them to any appointments or offering to negotiate on their behalf.

Of course the state sometimes discriminates in favour of older people. Think of free bus passes, free television licences and winter fuel payments, (at the moment!)

How can you tell if your friend is being abused?

Common signs and symptoms of any form of abuse displayed by an elderly person include anxiety, agitation, withdrawal, fear of being left alone and sleeplessness. Your elderly friend might start to show evidence of low self-esteem or a fear of new situations. Self-harm, an anxiety to please and subservience might also be observed.

If you notice that your friend has unexplained bruising, flinches as you pass or offers improbable explanations for injuries, it might be that they are covering up some sort of physical abuse.

An inexplicable shortage of money for day-to-day necessities, lack of food in the house, lack or disappearance of personal possessions, a cold house or non-payment of bills, may indicate some form of financial abuse.

People will react to abuse in different ways according to their character and life experience. However all types of abuse will cause some degree of emotional distress to the person abused and this will be shown in the individual's behaviour.

What can you do if you suspect your elderly friend is being abused?

Think carefully before you take any action. There might be a perfectly reasonable explanation for what is happening. Discuss your observations with your elderly friend to ascertain whether they feel they are being abused. Once you think that your suspicions are well founded, or if the signs of abuse are obvious, do not delay in reporting your concerns so that you can express them while the details are fresh in your memory. You can contact your local council adult protection team or, if your friend is in immediate danger, call the police who have workers trained to deal with suspected abuse. You can also use the helpline at Action on Elder Abuse – telephone: 08088088141 or seek help from Age UK, Mind or The Alzheimer's Society. Keep information confidential and do not tell other people about what you have seen or suspect unless they have a right to know.

BE A GOOD FRIEND

I think that it would be wise to remember that for some people getting old is not easy. How the body ages depends in part on family genes but lifestyle choices also have an impact. Over time it becomes harder to hear, visual sharpness declines, physical strength decreases and lapses of memory occur. The effects of aging might be loss of confidence or frustration at no longer being able to pursue hobbies and partake in activities. Deteriorating sight and hearing can result in isolation, leading to boredom. I must stress here that these changes are not inevitable.

Bear in mind that everyone, including your friend, has certain rights in laws that emanate from the United Nations Universal Declaration of Human Rights. For example, we all have the right to life, freedom of thought and expression, respect for individuality and privacy and access to information about ourselves held by other people. All this is too formal for what is mainly an informal situation. Rather I have taken the approach of asking what in a modern, decent society, should an elderly person living at home reasonably expect of an unpaid friend or relative acting as a carer?

To do this I have read through the Care Quality Commission's essential standards of care and have selected, paraphrased or expanded those that I think are relevant to the circumstances of a voluntary carer of an elderly friend. I put them forward as suggestions for you to consider.

Speak as you would wish to be spoken to

Treat your friend with respect at all times. Address them politely, give them chance to talk and listen to what they have to say. Above all, do not bully, swear at, ignore, tease, ridicule, embarrass or intimidate them.

Treat with dignity

Do not speak to your friend in a patronizing way, as if to a child. Rather address them as a responsible adult, consult them about their needs and wishes. Respect their views and take them into account even if they do not coincide with your own. My aunt habitually changes into her nightclothes at around 4 o'clock in the afternoon before, as she says, she gets too tired to bother. We might consider this behaviour to be socially bizarre but I respect her decision.

Respect privacy

It is particularly important to respect the privacy of your friend when they are dressing, undressing, bathing or going to the toilet. Knock on the door and ask permission to enter their room or home before doing so. Allow your friend time and space without the disturbance and intrusion of other people, including you, if that is what they wish. Neither my father nor my aunt appreciates having to receive visitors while their favourite programmes are on television. Being alone is not necessarily to be lonely although most elderly people are happy to have company.

Confidentiality

Confidentiality is about information. What you observe about a person or what a person tells you should not be passed on to other people. Of course within a family there may not be much information that is not already common knowledge. But as a general rule I suggest that, while caring for your friend, confidential information about them, such as their medical or financial circumstances, ought not to be passed on to any other person without your friends explicit consent.

Encourage individuality

Who would not agree that in principle an elderly person should be allowed to choose how they wish to live? For example, they should decide how to conduct their social life and the routines of daily living such as what and when to eat, when to go to bed and get up and what to wear. My father's idea of a sunny afternoon's enjoyment, is sitting in his garden wearing a straw sun hat, trousers rolled up over his knees and in his vest with a pistol at his side. These choices might not fit in with my idea of how to enjoy the sunshine, but people must be allowed, as far as is reasonably possible, to live as they choose. And the pistol? It was a water pistol – he hates cats in his garden.

As they get older and tired, confused or ill your elderly friend may wish to be looked after, asking you to make decisions on their behalf. I remember such a friend who was not at all interested in maintaining her independence, although physically able, she preferred others to make decisions for her. Another person might insist on their right to make their own decisions.

Maintaining independence

I suggest that you should encourage your friend to remain independent as it is good for their self-respect. You can help with the decision-making by offering advice and proposing alternatives. I discussed with my father his increasing difficulty in dressing himself because of the buttons on his shirt and having to pull his jersey over his head. After some initial reluctance, he changed his dress to T-shirts and cardigans. The solution has allowed him to maintain a degree of independence and saved him from the distress of being unable to manage unaided.

Where there is a conflict between their wishes and what you think are their best interests, discuss the problem with your friend, using explanations, persuasion and encouragement to help them make their own decisions.

Different cultures and values

If your friend is of a different social, cultural or religious background from yourself, you can show your respect and support, by being tolerant of their way of life. Encourage them to maintain their social, political and religious affiliations. Don't forget, people who are old are as different from each other as you and I are.

CARING FOR THE CARER

Do not forget that you too have needs, so do not let your elderly friend determine for how long and how frequently you spend time with them.

Who is a carer?

I have used the Carers UK definition as people who 'provide unpaid care by looking after an elderly, ill, frail or disabled family member, friend or partner'. Many organizations that provide support for older people publish free leaflets about the various forms of help available for carers, including discussion forums, advice lines and local support groups.

It would be wise to remember that as a volunteer **you** choose how much care and time you are prepared to give. However, once you accept payment, the person for whom you are providing the care will feel justified in defining the care they need and the amount of time you spend with them.

For those of us who are not angels

Although it is usual for a wife or husband to look after their partner, for many people it is something they do out of a sense of duty and compassion. Others may feel that it has become their responsibility to care for an elderly relative or friend, for example, an only child, the youngest daughter, the son or daughter living nearby. I therefore include some ideas that may help them to clarify their attitudes to caring and to help them stay positive, tolerant, and good-humoured towards those for whom they care.

Care for yourself first, because unless you do, you will not be able to care for someone else. Make efforts to maintain your own lifestyle by taking time to take care of yourself, do the things you enjoy and meet your own friends for a light-hearted chat. You will then feel better able to be patient and tolerant of the person for whom you are caring.

Set limits on the type and amount of care you give and take breaks from the responsibility of caring without feeling guilty. Don't feel that you have to say "yes" to every request. Expect to be treated with consideration by your friend and to be spoken to politely and in a kindly manner.

Remember, you cannot expect the person you are caring for to become the person you would like them to be, or to do what you would like them to do. They are not there to fulfil your expectations of what growing older should be like. Accept that, despite all your efforts, your friend is probably going to need more care rather than less care as they become older.

Try not to be hard on yourself if you cannot make someone's life all that you or they would want it to be. You may find this is difficult if you are emotionally attached to the person for whom you are caring.

People who can help

If you feel that it is getting hard for you to cope alone, for example, if you are not getting enough sleep, your family relationships are suffering or your work commitments are being compromised, make contact with the local authority's social services department. They will be able to put you in touch with any respite care and adult day-care facilities in your area. As little as two hours respite, three times a week can make a big difference to how you cope and for how long you can continue to cope as a carer.

If someone else offers to help you to care for your friend, take advantage of the offer. If you make your needs known, you may be surprised by the willingness of friends and family members to lend a hand.

Carers groups are usually a good source of information and advice. You can probably find out who and where they are by enquiring at your local library, resource centre or doctor's surgery. Some organizations such as the Alzheimer's Society have local groups that arrange discussion sessions for carers and joint music therapy for both carers and their elderly friends.

Gov.uk is an internet site that provides information on public services such as benefits, jobs, pensions and health services. The web address is www.gov.uk

The following organizations might be able to offer help.

- Age UK is the new organization combining Age Concern and Help the Aged. Its advice line is: 0800 169 6565 and the website address is www.ageuk.org.uk

- In Wales you can contact Age Cymru: 0800 022 3444 or www.agecymru.org.uk

- In Scotland you can contact Age Scotland: 0800 470 8090 or www.agescotland.org.uk

- In Northern Ireland you can contact Age NI: 0808 808 7575 or www.ageni.org.uk

Carers Direct offers help and support if you want to talk to someone about your caring role and the options available to you. You can write to PO Box 4338 Manchester, M61 0BY, telephone 0300 123 1053 or visit www.nhs.uk/carersdirect

Carers UK provides information and support for carers including information about benefits. To contact the organization write to 20 Great Dover Street, London, SE1 4LX. You can also call Careline on 0808 808 7777 or visit www.carersuk.org

Citizens Advice Bureau (CAB) is a national network of advice centres offering free, confidential and independent advice through their local centres, or visit www.citizensadvice.org.uk

The Princess Royal Trust for Carers and Crossroads Care are now known as Carers Trust and is a nationwide organization operating over 140 Carers' Centres that provide information and advice. Its Head Office is at 32-36 Loman Street, London, SE1 0EH and it can be contacted at www.carers.org or on 0844 800 4361. It has a local centre in many towns, but not all, throughout the UK.

WHAT HAPPENS NEXT?

After maybe years of caring for your friend one day they die and you are left to grieve, with a big hole in your life and an unusual amount of spare time. You are supposed to be relieved that the caring role is over, but that is not always how it feels.

Do not allow yourself to spend too much time in going over what more you could have perhaps done or how differently you could have behaved. It is probably not possible to behave at all times as you would like to and to be always patient and good-humoured.

Allow yourself time to recover and to pick up on the social life you might have compromised whilst caring. When you feel ready, make the effort. I think I shall keep chickens in my garden! The habit of caring will be hard to break.

For help and advice on grieving, Age UK have published a booklet available online at ageuk.org.uk

Cruse Bereavement Care is a counselling and advice service for bereaved people and also offers advice, information and practical support, telephone 0844 477 9400 or visit www.cruse.org.uk

ABOUT THE AUTHOR

As a young woman I completed my nurse training at Manchester Royal Infirmary and worked in general, paediatrics and community nursing until I married. After that a family of three children soon sprang into being and so put my career on hold for several years. When the children had grown to a responsible age, if they ever do, I resumed my career, accepting a post at a nearby nursing home, eventually becoming the manager. I introduced a programme of work based training. After six years I accepted the post of the Training Manager with a mission to introduce quality care training into all the company's homes. It was a challenging but enjoyable experience. I have now retired from that position to enjoy the company of my six grandchildren and to commit damage to the fairways of the local golf courses.

I was prompted to write this book as for the past few years I have been caring for my elderly father and my less elderly aunt, living in their own homes in the village where I live.

Towards the end of writing this book, my father celebrated his century with a splendid party for all his family and friends. He took a great deal of pleasure from the company of his great-grandchildren who, at the party, formed a band to play music for him. He died shortly before his 101st birthday.

www.ingramcontent.com/pod-product-compliance
Ingram Content Group UK Ltd.
Pitfield, Milton Keynes, MK11 3LW, UK
UKHW021829070325
4898UKWH00042B/939